MW01077343

POLE DANCING TO GOSPEL HYMNS

BY ANDREA GIBSON

A Write Bloody Book
Long Beach. CA USA

Pole Dancing to Gospel Hymns
by Andrea Gibson

Write Bloody Publishing ©2008–2010.
2nd Edition.
Printed in USA

Pole Dancing to Gospel Hymns Copyright 2008–2010.
All Rights Reserved.

Published by Write Bloody Publishing.

Printed in Long Beach, CA USA.

Cover Designed by Jeff Harmon
Photo by Drew Angerer
Illustrations by Anis Mojgani
Interior Layout by Lea C. Deschenes
Edited by Saadia Byram and Derrick Brown
Type set in Helvetica Neue and Bell MT

To contact the author, send an email to writebloody@gmail.com

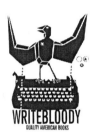

WRITE BLOODY PUBLISHING
LONG BEACH, CA

"I wish I'd a knowed more people. I would have loved 'em all. If I'd a knowed more I'd a loved more."

—From Toni Morrison's *Song of Solomon*

For Vox Feminista,
"Comforting the disturbed
and disturbing the comfortable."
Enormous Thanks.

www.voxfeminista.org

POLE DANCING TO GOSPEL HYMNS

POLE DANCER

She pole-dances to gospel hymns.
Came out to her family in the middle of Thanksgiving grace.
I knew she was trouble
two years before our first date.
But my heart was a Labrador Retriever
with its head hung out the window of a car
tongue flapping in the wind
on a highway going 95
whenever she walked by.

So I mastered the art of crochet
and I crocheted her a winter scarf
and one night at the bar I gave it to her with a note
that said something like,
I hope this keeps your neck warm.
If it doesn't give me a call.

The key to finding love
is fucking up the pattern on purpose,
is skipping a stitch,
is leaving a tiny, tiny hole to let the cold in
and hoping she mends it with your lips.

This morning I was counting her freckles.
She has five on the left side of her face, seven on the other
and I love her for every speck of trouble she is.
She's frickin' awesome.
Like popcorn at a drive-in movie
that neither of us has any intention of watching.
Like Batman and Robin
in a pick-up truck in the front row with the windows steamed up.

Like Pacman in the eighties,
she swallows my ghosts.

Slaps me on my dark side and says,
"Baby, this is the best day ever."
So I stop listening for the sound of the ocean
in the shells of bullets I hoped missed us
to see there are white flags from the tips of her toes
to her tear ducts
and I can wear her halos as handcuffs
'cause I don't wanna be a witness to this life,
I want to be charged and convicted,
ear lifted to her song like a bouquet of *yes*
because my heart is a parachute that has never opened in time
and I wanna fuck up that pattern,
leave a hole where the cold comes in and fill it every day with her sun,
'cause anyone who has ever sat in lotus for more than a few seconds
knows it takes a hell of a lot more muscle to stay than to go.

And I want to grow
strong as the last patch of sage on a hillside
stretching towards the lightning.
God has always been an arsonist.
Heaven has always been on fire.
She is a butterfly knife bursting from a cocoon in my belly.
Love is a half moon hanging above Baghdad
promising to one day grow full,
to pull the tides through our desert wounds
and fill every clip of empty shells with the ocean.
Already there is salt on my lips.

Lover, this is not just another poem.
This is my goddamn revolt.
I am done holding my tongue like a bible.
There is too much war in every verse of our silence.
We have all dug too many trenches away from ourselves.

This time I want to melt like a snowman in Georgia,
'til my smile is a pile of rocks you can pick up
and skip across the lake of your doubts.

Trust me,
I have been practicing my ripple.
I have been breaking into mannequin factories
and pouring my pink heart into their white paint.
I have been painting the night sky upon the inside of doorframes
so only moonshine will fall on your head in the earthquake.
I have been collecting your whispers and your whiplash
and your half–hour-long voice mail messages.
Lover, did you see the sunset tonight?
Did you see Neruda lay down on the horizon?
Do you know it was his lover who painted him red,
who made him stare down the bullet holes
in his country's heart?

I am not looking for roses.
I want to break like a fever.
I want to break like the Berlin Wall.
I want to break like the clouds
so we can see every fearless star,
how they never speak *guardrail*,
how they only say *fall*.

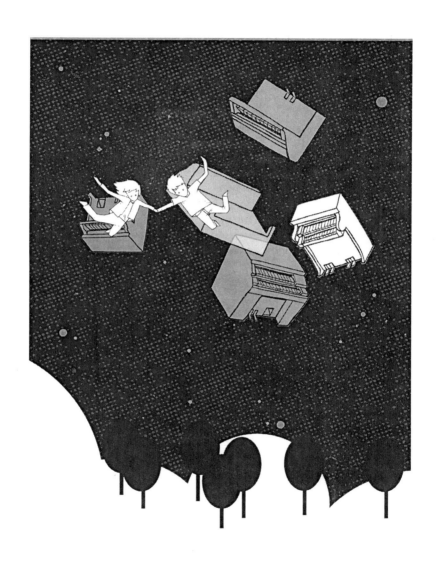

YARROW

We packed our lives into the back of your truck
and drove two thousand miles
back to the only home you'd ever known.
On the bayou you ate crawfish.
I wished I had never become a vegetarian.

Here, whatever you came carrying
fell to the ground like Creole swamp rain.
Uptown you could watch the jazz notes float
from porch swings to sidewalks of little girls
playing jump rope and hopscotch,
to old women skipping rocks
across the gulf of the Mississippi
like heartbeats they forgot they had,
while mid-city trombones
wrote love poems in lonely men's ears.

For a year we were gardeners.
"No, Andrea, yarrow doesn't grow here,
imagine a womb full of water,
plant like you would plant a daughter,
name her Iris, Rose, Magnolia, and Gardenia."

You could hold the soil between your fingers
and smell gumbo and harmonicas.
Could smell po-boys and cathedrals on the same block.

"What do ya mean, you don't talk to strangers?
Come inside and see a picture of my son,
he raises hell, but he's a good one…"
Iris, Rose, Magnolia, Gardenia,

when I heard of Katrina
I thought, "The flowers, save the flowers…"

I never thought for a second
we wouldn't save the people.

BIRTHDAY

For Jenn

At 12 years old I started bleeding with the moon
and began beating up boys who dreamed of becoming astronauts.
I fought with my knuckles white as dust,
and left bruises the shape of Salem.
There are things we know by heart.
And things we don't.

At 13 my friend Jen tried to teach me how to blow rings of smoke.
I'd watch the nicotine rising from her lips like fading halos,
but I could never make dying beautiful.

The sky didn't fill with colors the night I convinced myself
veins are kite strings you can only cut free.
I suppose I love this life,

in spite of my clenched fist.

I open my palm and my lifelines look like branches from an Aspen tree,
and there are songbirds perched on the tips of my fingers,

and I wonder if Beethoven held his breath
the first time his fingers touched the keys
the same way a soldier holds his breath
the first time his finger coaxes the trigger.
We all have different reasons for forgetting to breathe.

My lungs remember
the day my mother took my hand and placed it on her belly
and told me the symphony beneath was my baby sister's heartbeat.
and her lungs were taking shape

And I knew life would tremble
like the first tear on a prison guard's unturned cheek,
like a stumbling prayer on a dying man's lips,
like a vet holding a full bottle of whisky
as if it were an empty gun in a war zone…
just take me   just take me

Sometimes the scales themselves weigh far too much,
the heaviness of forever balancing blue sky with red blood.
We were all born on days when too many people died in terrible ways,
but you still have to call it a *birth*day.
You still have to fall for the prettiest girl on the playground at recess
and hope she knows you can hit a baseball
further than any boy in the whole third grade

and I've been running for home
through the windpipe of a man who sings
while his hands play washboard with a spoon
on a street corner in New Orleans
where every boarded-up window is still painted with the words
We're Coming Back
like a promise to the ocean
that we will always keep moving towards the music,
the way Basquiat slept in a cardboard box to be closer to the rain.

Beauty, catch me on your tongue.
Thunder, clap us open.
The pupils in our eyes were not born to hide beneath their desks.
Tonight, lay us down to rest in the Arizona desert,
then wake us to wash the feet of pregnant women
who climbed across the border with their bellies aimed towards the sun.
I know a thousand things louder than a soldier's gun.

I know the heartbeat of his mother.

There is a boy writing poems in Central Park
and as he writes he moves
and his bones become the bars of Mandela's jail cell stretching apart,
and there are men playing chess in the December cold
who can't tell if the breath rising from the board
is their opponents' or their own,
and there's a woman on the stairwell of the subway
swearing she can hear Niagara Falls from her rooftop in Brooklyn,
and I'm remembering how Niagara Falls is a city overrun
with strip-malls and traffic and vendors
and *one* incredibly brave river that makes it all worth it.

I know this world is far from perfect.
I am not the type to mistake a streetlight for the moon.
I know our wounds are deep as the Atlantic.
But every ocean has a shoreline
and every shoreline has a tide
that is constantly returning
to wake the songbirds in our hands,
to wake the music in our bones,
to place one fearless kiss on the mouth of that new born river
that has to run through the center of our hearts
to find its way home.

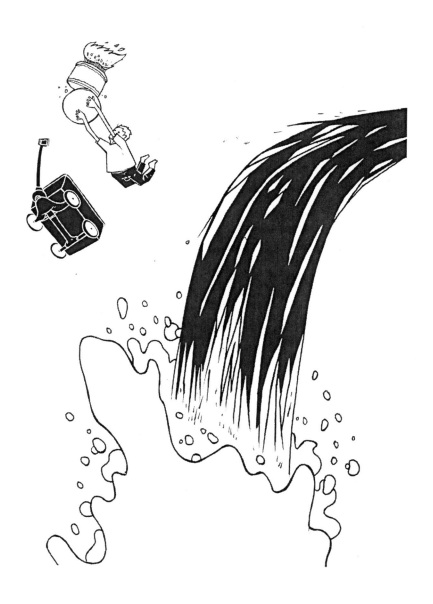

FOR ELI

Eli came back from Iraq
and tattooed a teddy bear onto the inside of his wrist.
Above that a medic with an IV bag,
above that an angel
but Eli says the teddy bear won't live.

And I know I don't know but I say, "I know."
'Cause Eli's only twenty-four and I've never seen eyes
further away from childhood than his,
eyes old with a wisdom
he knows I'd rather not have.

Eli's mother traces a teddy bear onto the inside of my arm
and says, "Not all casualties come home in body bags."

And I swear,
I'd spend the rest of my life writing nothing
but the word *light* at the end of this tunnel
if I could find the fucking tunnel
I'd write nothing but white flags.

Somebody pray for the soldiers.
Somebody pray for what's lost.
Somebody pray for the mailbox
that holds the official letters
to the mothers, fathers,
sisters and little brothers
of Michael 19... Steven 21... John 33.
How ironic that their deaths sound like bible verses.

The hearse is parked in the halls of the high school
recruiting black, brown and poor

while anti-war activists outside Walter Reed Army Hospital
scream, "100,000 slain,"
as an amputee on the third floor
breathes forget-me-nots onto the window pane.
But how can we forget what we never knew?

Our sky is so perfectly blue it's repulsive.
Somebody tell me where god lives
'cause if god is truth, god doesn't live here.
Our lies have seared the sun too hot to live by.
There are ghosts of kids who are still alive
toting M16s with trembling hands
while we dream ourselves stars on Survivor,
another missile sets fire to the face in the locket
of a mother whose son needed money for college
and she swears she can feel his photograph burn.

How many wars will it take us to learn
that only the dead return?
The rest remain forever caught between worlds of
shrapnel shatters body of three-year-old girl
to…
welcome to McDonalds, can I take your order?

The mortar of sanity crumbling,
stumbling back home to a home that will never be home again.
Eli doesn't know if he can ever write a poem again.
One third of the homeless men in this country are veterans.
And we have the nerve to *Support Our Troops*
with pretty yellow ribbons
while giving nothing but dirty looks to their outstretched hands.

Tell me, what land of the free
sets free its eighteen-year-old kids into greedy war zones
hones them like missiles
then returns their bones in the middle of the night
so no one can see?

Each death swept beneath the carpet and hidden like dirt,
each life a promise we never kept.

Jeff Lucey came back from Iraq
and hung himself in his parents' basement with a garden hose.
The night before he died he spent forty-five minutes on his father's lap
rocking like a baby,
rocking like *daddy, save me,*
and don't think for a minute he too isn't collateral damage
in the mansions of Washington.
They are watching them burn and hoarding the water.
Which senators' sons are being sent out to slaughter?
Which presidents' daughters are licking ashes from their lips
or dreaming up ropes to wrap around their necks
in case they ever make it home alive?

Our eyes are closed, America.
There are souls in the boots of the soldiers, America.
Fuck your yellow ribbon.
You wanna support our troops,
bring them home,
and hold them tight when they get here.

ANYTHING

Tonight I'd swear the man in the moon is a rapist,
and stars are nothing but scars,
bullet wounds from humanity's drive-by
firing at the face of the sky.
Tonight crying would be too easy.
It would please me too much
and no I don't want you to touch me
'cause your hands are clean
and I'm filthy,
guilty with the blood of something beautiful all over me.

I've been weak and leaking so much poison
in all the rivers around me the fish are dying,
and the trees are vying for some light
but I'm the eternal night
writing rhymes about wind chimes and world peace
while even in my sleep I'm fighting wars
that grind the enamel off my teeth
and I wake with my jaw clenched and my body bent
thinking, "How many dishes have I broken this week?"
in an attempt to not break myself
by taking brutal belt to my hide
'cause it's hard to wanna survive.

And all the great therapists of this world might say,
"Maybe your anger is good.
Maybe your rage is you emerging from the cage
of everything you've been."
So I try to be Zen, singing mantras of
om mani padme hum
but god fears me too much to hear me,

and my heart beats another kid in the candy store
and his mother calls the cops
and every time the clock ticks
I start tick tick tick talking more shit,
my voice sounding the crucifixion of everything holy.
There are blisters on my tongue
from pounding nails into hearts of prophets,
and just when I think I can stop it
satan resurrects inside me
and everything around me turns to hell.
Last night I stole pennies from a wishing well
to buy rope to lynch the last inch of hope from the planet
and all…

because you have a new girlfriend and I can't stand it.

I wanted to be eighty together,
wanted to birth poems like babies together
and watch them grow up to save the world.

'Cause girl, you're the only one
who could ever raise the sun inside me.
And I swear the ground beneath my feet
is only soft because you walk beside.
There were times I thought I was so lost
even god would never find me
and then you came up right behind me
and kissed a cross onto my back.

And it's things like that that got me going crazy,
'cause I was thinking maybe the breaths we'd take together
would make us live forever,
and now you're killing me.
Look at me, I'm dying,
not even trying to evolve when
I wanted to be there forty years from now

when the doctor called to say
your mother might not make it another day.
And I wasn't gonna be just ok.
I was gonna be perfect.

Was gonna make my love feel
like the first time you rode your bike without training wheels,
kneel before you every day
like there was no one else before you,
'cause I've heard your heart beat
like that breeze that could bring any violence to its knees
and the best lines I've ever written…

I plagiarized every word from the thoughts of yours I heard
while you were just sitting in silence,
staring up at Mars
but you never wish on shooting stars
you wish on the ones
that have the courage to shine where they are,
no matter how dark the night.

And how now do I turn away from that light
when I wanted to be eighty with you,
birth babies like poems with you
and let them write themselves.

Was gonna hold your heart to my ear like a seashell
'til I could hear the tides of every tear you've ever cried,
then build islands in the seas of your eyes
so you'd see there's land to swim to.
Hold your hand and say, "Storms are born
from the same sky we write hymns to when the sun shines.
Sometimes it takes tempests to wake rainbows
that will wind our pain into halos."

Was gonna carve your name into my wrist
so my pulse could kiss you.

Was gonna love you so well
I'd wake every morning
and tell you things like this,
"Bliss is the moments you're with me
when you're gone my life hurts like hell
but I'll do anything to make you happy
even if it means setting you free
to be with someone else."

SWING-SET

"Are you a boy or a girl?" he asks,
staring up from all three feet
of his pudding-faced grandeur.

I say, "Dylan, you've been in this class for three years
and you still don't know if I'm a boy or a girl?"

"Uh-uh."

"Well then, at this point I really don't think it matters, do you?"

"Um... no. Can I have a push on the swing?"

And this happens every day.
It's a tidal wave of kindergarten curiosity
rushing straight for the rocks of me,
whatever I am.

In the classroom we discuss the milky way galaxy,
the orbit of the sun around the earth or... whatever.
Jupiter! Saturn! Mars!
"Kids, do you know that some of the stars
we see up in the sky are so far away they've already burned out?
What do you think of that...Timmy?"

"Um...my mom says that even though you've got
hairs that grow from your legs
and the hairs on your head grow short and pokey
and you smell really bad like my dad
that you're a girl."

"You're right. Thank you, Timmy."

And so it goes.
On the playground she stares up
from behind her pink powder puff sunglasses
and asks, "Do you have a boyfriend?"

"No."

"Ohhh" she says. "Do you have a girlfriend?"

I say, "No, but if by some miracle twenty years from now
I ever finally do, I'll definitely bring her by to meet you.
How's that?"

"OK...can I have push on the swing?"

And that's the thing.
They don't care.
They don't care.
We, on the other hand...
My father sitting across the table at Christmas dinner
gritting his teeth over his still-full plate
his appetite raped away
by the intrusion of my haircut,
"What were you thinking? You used to be such a pretty girl!"

Frat boys drunk and screaming
leaning out the windows of their daddies' SUVs
"Hey, are you a faggot or a dyke?!"
And I wonder what would happen
if I met up with them in the middle of the night.

Then of course there's always the not-quite-bright-enough
fluorescent light of the public restroom,
"Sir! Sir! Do you realize this is the ladies' room?!"

"Yes, ma'am, I do.
It's just I didn't feel comfortable
sticking this tampon up my penis
in the men's room."

But the best is always the mother at the market,
sticking up her nose
while pushing aside her child's wide eyes
whispering, "Don't stare, it's rude."

And I wanna say, "Listen, lady,
the only rude thing I see
is your paranoid, parental hand
pushing aside the best education on *self*
that little girl's ever gonna get
living with your Maybelline lips, Stair Master hips
synthetic, kiwi, vanilla 'spilling beauty.
So why don't you take your pinks and blues,
your boy-girl rules
and shove 'em in that cart
with your fucking issue of Cosmo,
'cause tomorrow
I start my day with twenty-eight minds
that know a hell of a lot more than you do,
and if I show up in a pink frilly dress
those kids won't love me any more or less."

"Hey... are you a boy or a... oh, never mind,
can I have a push on the swing?"

And someday,
when we grow up,
it's all gonna be that simple.

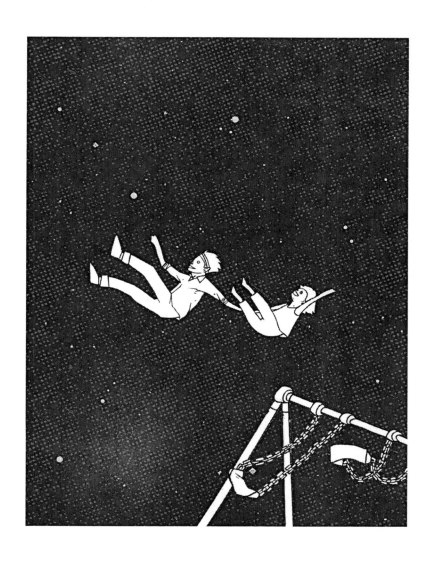

TADPOLES

A tadpole doesn't know
it's gonna grow bigger.
It just swims,
and figures limbs
are for frogs.

People don't know
the power they hold.
They just sing hymns,
and figure saving
is for god.

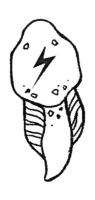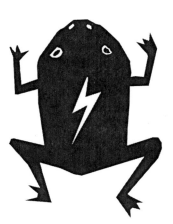

BLUE BLANKET

Still there are days when there is no way,
not even a chance,
that I'd dare for even a second
glance at the reflection of my body in the mirror
and she knows why.

Like I know why she only cries
when she feels like she's about to lose control.
She knows how much control is worth,
knows what a woman can lose when her power to move
is taken away

by a grip so thick with hate
it could clip the wings of Isis,
leave the next eight generations of your blood shaking.

And tonight
something inside me is breaking,

my heart beating so deep beneath the sheets of her pain
I could give every tear she's crying a year, a name,
and a face I'd forever erase from her mind if I could.

But how much closer to free would any of us be
if even a few of us forgot
what too many women in this world cannot.
And I'm thinking, "What the hell would you tell your daughter?"
Your someday daughter
when you'd have to hold her beautiful face
to the beat up face of this place
that hasn't learned the meaning of
STOP.

What would you tell your daughter of the womb raped empty,
the eyes swollen shut,
the gut too frightened to hold food,
the thousands upon thousands of bodies used?

It was seven minutes of the worst kind of hell.
Seven.
And she stopped believing in heaven.

distrust became her law,
fear her bible,
the only chance of survival…
don't trust any of them.

Bolt the doors to your home,
iron gate your windows,
walking to your car alone
get the keys in the lock
please please please please open
like already you can feel
that five-fingered noose around your neck
two hundred pounds of hatred
digging graves into the sacred soil of your flesh
please please please please open
already you're choking for your breath
listening for the broken record of the defense,
Answer the question,
Answer the question.
Answer the question, miss!

Why am I on trial for this?
Would you talk to your daughter,
your sister, your mother like this?
I am generations of daughters, sisters, mothers,
our bodies battlefields, war grounds
beneath the weapons of your brothers' hands.

Do you know they've found landmines
in broken women's souls?
Black holes in the parts of their hearts
that once sang symphonies of creation
bright as the light on infinity's halo.

She says, "I remember the way love
used to glow on my skin
before he made his way in
now every touch feels like a sin
that could crucify Medusa, Kali, Oshun, Mary
bury me in a blue blanket so their god doesn't know I'm a girl,
cut off my curls,
I want peace when I'm dead."
Her friend knocks at the door,
"It's been three weeks,
don't you think it's time you got out of bed?"
"No, the ceiling fan still feels like his breath,
I think I need just a couple more days of rest, please."

Bruises on her knees from praying to forget.
She's heard stories of Vietnam vets
who can still feel the tingling of their amputated limbs.
She's wondering how many women are walking around this world
feeling the tingling of their amputated wings,
remembering what it was to fly, to sing.

Tonight she's not wondering
what she would tell her daughter.
She knows what she would tell her daughter.
She'd ask her, "What gods do you believe in?
I'll build you a temple of mirrors so you can see them.
Pick the brightest star you've ever wished on.
I'll show you the light in you
that made that wish come true..."

Tonight she's not asking you what you would tell your daughter.
She's life deep in the hell, the slaughter,
has already died a thousand deaths with every unsteady breath,
a thousand graves in every pore of her flesh
and she knows the war's not over,
knows there's bleeding to come,
knows she's far from the only woman or girl
trusting this world no more than the hands
trust rusted barbed wire.

She was whole before that night.
Believed in heaven before that night,
and she's not the only one.
She knows she won't be the only one.
She's not asking what you're gonna tell your daughter.
She asking what you're gonna teach
your son.

LOVE POEM

You
are the music of two grasshoppers
making love in a school yard
where four-year-olds ask me,
what are the grasshoppers doing?
and I tell them they're dancing to the music of
You
are the gaps in my ribcage
where the sunrise winds through to my heart and
You
are the part of the sunset that is so pink
the grasshoppers think maybe we should stop and watch
You
are the moon when it bloomed for the very first time
and a child inspired unwound the lid of a jar
that set ten-thousand grasshoppers free and
You
drive me fucking crazy.

I mean insanely.
You make me wanna take a fork to my eyeballs,
rip the hair from my armpits
and shove it down my throat
'cause I would rather choke
than argue another minute with you
but you are so

pretty.

And smart.
You know so many words.
You're every poem I would write

if ink could ever hold the light
that glows from your toes
when you're climbing up trees.
Girl, I swear ya got sap running thick in your veins
and I never love you more
than when you're mourning the death of raindrops
falling forsaken on pavement.
God, I love how you hate pavement.

But you make me wanna smash my skull on pavement.
It's true.
When we argue you make me wanna rip off my nose,
bone and all like my uncle Billy used to pretend to do.
He'd say, "Girl, I'm gonna rip off yer nose!"
Then he'd tug at my face
and hold up half his thumb
and half the time he'd fool me and I'd start crying.
But I'm older now and I'm not lying
you make me wanna rip off my nose.

Except when you don't.
Sometimes you make me wish I had an extra nose
only to smell your hair,
because I love how your hair smells like... hair.
I always hated the smell of shampoo,
Besides
I love you.
It's true.

The way you pretend to chew gum when you're nervous.
The way you stick out your tongue
when you look in the mirror
'cause you think your face is shaped better that way.
And I love the way you pray
and I love the way you chew
and use chopsticks like you're from Japan.

God, you're a woman of culture.
I wanna eat you like a... not a vulture

a swan.

I wanna eat you like swans eat flowers.
Baby, if swans ever ate flowers
I would eat you like that for hours.

Except when you're sour
and acting like a self-righteous grumpy old grump
like ya do sometimes,
'cause those times
you make me wanna run to the edge of the fucking world
and hurl myself into a black fucking hole
and never come back ever.

And then there're the times I wanna
be with you forever and follow you forever
wherever you go
if only for the freckle in the middle of your belly
that's just like mine,
or the time you corrected me for saying *man*
instead of *human kind*.
I can't believe I did that.

Do you know how much I love your boobs?
Almost as much as I love how
you hate that I call breasts *boobs*
and say you're tired of dating a 12-year-old boy,
but god, your boobs bring me joy.
Though I could live forever between the lines of your teeth
and eat nothing but memory and purge myself clean.

You are a dream.
We are a nightmare sometimes.

But if you wake up terrified
I'll be there to hold you,
fold you in the pockets of my faith
and say, "We'll be ok."

HOOK LINE

There are stars in your dark side
brighter than the sun.

Promise me, if you ever catch your breath
you will throw it back out to sea immediately.

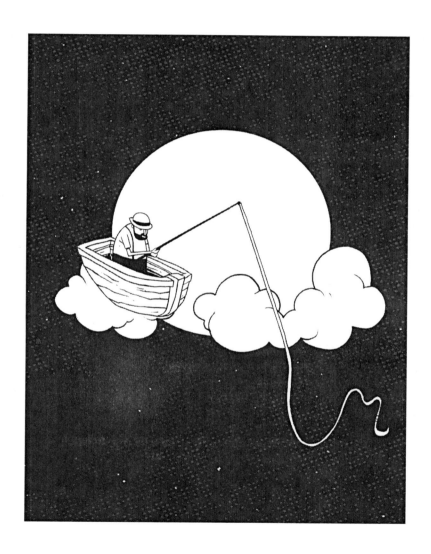

DIVE

.

Life doesn't rhyme.
It's bullets... and wind chimes.
It's lynchings... and birthday parties.
It's the rope that ties the noose
and the rope that hangs the backyard swing.

It's wanting tonight to speak the most honest poem
I've ever spoken in my life
not knowing if that poem should bring you closer
to living or dying.

Last night I prayed myself to sleep,
woke this morning to find god's obituary
scrolled in tears on my sheets
then walked outside to hear my neighbor
erasing ten thousand years of hard labor
with a single note of his violin
and the sound of the traffic rang like a hymn
as the holiest leaf of autumn
fell from a plastic tree limb, beautiful
and ugly.

Like right now I'm needing nothing more than for you to hug me
and if you do I'm gonna scream like a caged bird.
Life doesn't rhyme.
Sometimes love is a vulgar word.

I've heard saints preaching truths
that would have burned me at the stake.
I've heard poets telling lies that made me believe in heaven.

Sometimes I imagine Hitler at seven years old,
a paint brush in his hand at school
thinking, "What color should I paint my soul?"

Sometimes I remember myself
with track marks on my tongue
from shooting up convictions
that would have hung innocent men from trees.

Have you ever seen a mother falling to her knees
the day her son dies in a war she voted for?
Can you imagine how many gay teen-aged lives were saved
the day Matthew Shepard died?
Could there have been anything louder
than the noise inside his father's head
when he begged the jury, "Please don't take the lives
of the men who turned my son's skull to powder."
And I know nothing would make my family prouder
than if I gave up everything I believe in
but nothing keeps me believing
like the sound of my mother breathing.
Life doesn't rhyme.
It's tasting your rapist's breath
on the neck of a woman who loves you more
than anyone has loved you before
then feeling holy as Mary
beneath the hands of a one-night stand
who's calling somebody else's name.

It's you never feeling more greedy
than when you're handing out dollars to the needy.

It's my not eating meat for the last ten years
then seeing the kindest eyes I've ever seen in my life
on the face of a man with a branding iron in his hand
and a beat-down baby calf wailing at his feet.

It's choking on your beliefs.
It's your worst sin saving your fucking life.
It's the devil's knife carving holes into your soul
so angels will have a place to make their way inside.

Life doesn't rhyme.
Life is poetry, not math.
All the world's a stage
but the stage is a meditation mat.
You tilt your head back.
You breathe.
When your heart is broken you plant seeds in the cracks
and you pray for rain.
And you teach your sons and daughters
there are sharks in the water
but the only way to survive
is to breathe deep
and dive.

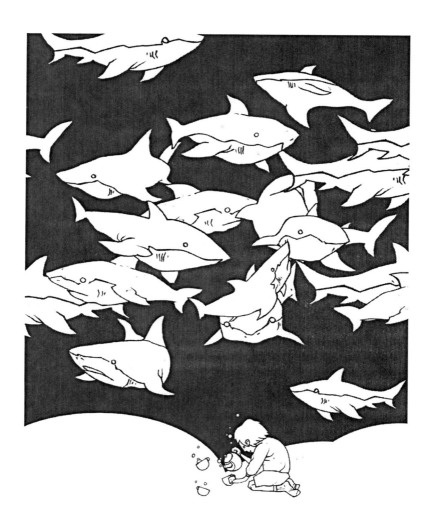

TITANIC

I grew up in the town that received the first distress signal
saying the Titanic was going down.
It was the only thing we were ever renowned for.
In fact, we prided ourselves on our failure to save the sinking
which is maybe part of the reason I prided myself
on drinking my first fifth of whisky at eleven years old.
It's cold where I come from.
I learned to drown young.

At fourteen I showed up to my 8 am high school art class so drunk
my art teacher took a month-long sabbatical to reevaluate
her ability to make the world a better place.
When she returned she had a face like a gravestone
with an already-passed death date.
I sometimes wonder if I killed her.

Which is maybe part of the reason
I sometimes paint this world prettier than it is.
Have you ever had the feeling you owe somebody somewhere
a really good reason to live?
To grow old?
To be ninety-eight-and-a-half
with a laugh like broken glass
so whenever folks walk barefoot
they'll get hidden pieces embedded in their souls?

I've spent too many years
sewing my tears together with thread
and hanging them like Christmas lights,
spent too many nights watching the sunset
on the edge of a knife's glint

to wanna let myself or anybody else drown anymore,
so call this poem shore
that when the message in the bottle finally arrives
it's not gonna ask what broke us in half,
it's gonna ask us why we survived.

Why did Rumi dance when his beloved died?
Why did children search Hiroshima's sky for the moon
when their wounds were still open as hope's suicide note,
when the clouds were still bleeding?
Why did Frida Kahlo sculpt a paintbrush from her scars?

My mother says the thing about wheelchairs
is they keep you looking up.
Says forests may be gorgeous
but there's nothing more alive
than a tree that grows in a cemetery
and sometimes it's the cup that's half empty
that fills the heart so full
it could pull a bow
above the strings of a row of combat boots
and make them sing like a pair of lovers calling each other's names
into the echo of the Grand Canyon.

Three years ago my niece's eyes
kept the needle from my sister's veins
for the very first time.
If I could collect that day,
the sweat from her shaking palms,
the cramps knotting like a noose in her gut
I would have the stuff of monarchs taking flight,
of nights when the smoke of burning flags
floats across our borders like a kiss.

It hit 170 degrees in the locked trailer of the truck
when the women locked hands and sang so hard

the Texas desert shook
like the hearts of the folks
who would find them still alive.

Why did Rumi dance?
We have cried so hard our tears have left scars on our cheekbones,
but who finds their way home by the short cuts?
You wrote your first song on a homophobe's fist.
She wrote her first poem on her mother's dying wish.

Sometimes the deepest breaths
are pulled from the bottom of the ocean floor,
and if the soul is a mosaic of all our broken pieces
I won't shine my rusted edges.
I'll just meet you on the shore.

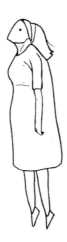

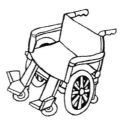

STAY

Stay.
There are snowflakes on my tongue
I want to melt on your inner thigh.
There's a face in the moon
I still call Jesus some nights.
My body is a temple where I've burned so many scriptures
I see smoke every time I look in the mirror.

Kiss me where the flames turned blue.
Tell me there are places on my skin
that look exactly like the sky
and your heart is a jet plane
heavy with the weight of businessmen and crying babies
but you're done running for the exit row.

'Cause god knows we have smoked the stars,
made wishes on falling ashes.
Something's gotta give,
it may as well be our fingers.
Touch me 'til my ribs become piano keys,
'til there is sheet music scrolled across the inside of my lungs
'cause I'm breaking old patterns.
For anyone else I would rhyme and end this line with saturn,
but you are not the type to wear rings,
and I'm not the type to want to celebrate forever
when Right Now is forever walking down the aisle unnoticed.

Hold me.
Sing me lullabies at dawn
when I've been up all night painting the wind
to remind myself that things are moving.

We were talking mountains and snowboards
when you said, "I'll teach you how to fall."

I said, "I bet you will."
But my bruises will be half-moons
hanging above corn fields
that grow only crop circles.
You are a mystery I promise I will never try to solve.
What science calls science I have always called miracle
and since we first met I have said "thank you" so many times
I have watched all of my broken pieces
curling into notes to plant themselves
in the soil of clarinets on street corners
in the French Quarter
you can find music
in places where you cannot find air.

So when you say you are homesick for my skin
my body sends you postcards from all its darkest corners
and prays you will still see the sun
climbing my bones like octaves,
'cause baby, there were nights when my pulse did not win,
nights when my heartbeat stained the kitchen floor bright red.
But you once told me
we are most alive in that split second before death,
so I call "ugly" a four letter word
and tell you I am tired of hearing myself swear.

Beauty
is in the eye of the beholder.
You hold me so well
that I am almost convinced
that smoke in the mirror
might one day disappear.

MARBLE

I once had sex with a very large woman
at the very very tip of a long quiet pier
while a herd of stranded sailors cheered us on
from a navy boat a hundred feet away
and that is just one of those things
I don't need to tell my mother.

But
there are other things I do need to tell her,
you, Mother.
'Cause I have been half a decade now
falling slow from the hands of your letting go,
crashing down upon the pages of our separation
where you've written me into paragraphs of
short-haired dirty-hippie man-hating queer.
And I wonder if you even remember my name.

'Cause every minute of every day
I can still hear you calling it from our window
through the wind of my ten-year-old sky,
"Andrea, it's time to come home…"

But I haven't been *home* in years.
And every memory of you is a halt,
a clot where all my blood-rushing veins just stop,
and most days I can't remember how to bleed.

But always, through it all
I have always breathed you
like the greatest breath I ever took.
The way I looked at you,

followed you in circles round the spiral
of your every single step, never missing a thing.

The way you would laugh, smile
sing me awake in the morning,
always crashing through my door without warning,
"Wake up, wake up, you sleepy head…"
And then you'd leave
as I pulled my tired body from the bed,
walked down the hall to find you
always in the middle of the living room
standing on your head,
your feet grinning at the ceiling, you'd say,
"Don't think so much, you're gonna suffocate your feelings.
Don't think so much, go out and play."

I remember the day I watched you carry
bucket after bucket of paint down the stairs
to our dark dingy basement.
Hours later you called me there to where you stood
pointing two dripping sticks at the once colorless walls.
"Look," you whispered.
"Fairies turned our basement to marble…"

And I marveled in you.
Always I marveled in you.
My mother,
rising from the ashes.
You were more than a phoenix.
You were the whole magnificent flock,
with your hundred thousand wings
shimmering light through the sky and I
wanted to be just like you.

But isn't it frightening what years will do
to even a spirit spun in the very velvet of song?

Isn't it frightening the way light will let go
of a heart that was once forever dancing,
releasing you now to the metal mold of constructed ideas
where fear somehow holding you from me
now folds you into terms
of Conservative Republican Christian,
while even Jesus knows
I was never born from any adjective,
I was born from you.

And I couldn't care less what you believe,
if only you would just believe in me,
'cause I am still carrying round our chord.
I am still shrouding myself in the lost chorus of your womb
hoping someday soon you will look and finally see me.

Look.
I am that little girl you held at three,
that almost-woman at seventeen.
I am that woman at sixty who will sit by your side
and hold your hand while you die.
I am that woman now.

And if you forever choose to shred the blankets of our blood
with the knives that hold our differences
we will both forever sleep cold.
But I will never forget the perfect warmth of you soul.
Will never forget my mother knew
that fairies danced on basement walls
and her song
the way she sang it when she woke me
would take me to a place
where feet could walk on ceilings
and feelings were always smarter things than thoughts.

And I am always
that woman's daughter.

TONIGHT

Offer your body as a burning building
without fire escapes.

I want to feel you like lifelines
on the palms of Christ
when the nails went through.

PHOTOGRAPH

I wish I was a photograph
tucked into the corners of your wallet,
a snapshot carried like a future in your back pocket.

I wish I was that face you show to strangers
when they ask you where you come from,
that someone that you come from
every time you get there,

and when you get there
I wish I was that someone who got phone calls
and postcards saying
wish you were here.

I wish you were here.
Autumn is the hardest season.
The leaves are all falling
and they're falling like they're falling in love with the ground
and the trees are naked and lonely.
I keep trying to tell them
new leaves will come around in the spring,
but you can't tell trees those things,
they're like me,
they just stand there
and don't listen.

I wish you were here.
I've been hazy-eyed
staring at the bottom of my glass again,
thinking of that time when it was so full
it was like we were tapping the moon for moonshine

or sticking straws into the center of the sun
and sipping like Icarus would forever kiss
the bullets from our guns.

I never meant to fire, you know.
I know you never meant to fire, lover.
Now the sky clicks from black to blue

and dusk looks like a bruise.

I've been wrapping one night stands
around my body like wedding bands
but none of them fit in the morning,
they just slip off my fingers and slip out the door
and all that lingers is the single scent of you.

Do you remember the night I told you
I've never seen anything more perfect than
than snow falling in the sodium glow of a street light,
electricity bowing to nature,
mind bowing to heartbeat,
This is gonna hurt bowing to *I love you.*
I still love you
like moons love the planets they circle around,
like children love recess bells,
I hear the sound of you
and think of playgrounds
where outcasts who stutter
beneath braces and bruises and acne
are finally learning that their rich handsome bullies
are never gonna grow up to be happy.
I think of happy when I think of you.

So wherever you are, I hope you're happy,
I really do.

I hope the stars are kissing your cheeks tonight.
I hope you finally found a way to quit smoking.
I hope your lungs are open and breathing this life.
I hope there's a kite in your hand
that's flying all the way up to Orion
and you still have a thousand yards of string to let out.
I hope you're smiling
like god is pulling at the corners of your mouth.

'Cause I might be naked and lonely,
shaking branches for bones,
but I'm still time zones away
from who I was the day before we met.
You were the first mile where my heart broke a sweat.
And I wish you were here.
I wish you'd never left.

THE YOGA INSTRUCTOR

When the yoga instructor broke Natalie's heart
she started hanging out at the Holocaust Museum
hoping to put her own pain into perspective.

On the phone I did not tell her
how I fell in love
the day George Bush was elected President,
and how I fell asleep that night
wrapped in the sweetest peace
I had ever known.

SEE THROUGH

We're on our way back to school from gymnastics class.
The kids are singing John Lennon's *Imagine*
at the back of the bus,
and only in Boulder, Colorado

Jesse stops herself mid-verse,
stretches her arm across the aisle like a sunbeam,
tugs at the hem of my shirt and asks,
"What does hatred mean?"

Jesse's five years old.
Anything I say, she's gonna believe.
But I realize I don't know the answers.
I don't know what hatred means.
I could guess and say it's the opposite of love.
I could guess and say,
"Jesse, hatred is wanting nothing but white faces
on our private-school bus."

But Jesse isn't white yet.
Go ahead and ask her.

"What color are you, Jesse?"

"Well, it looks like I'm pink."

Shane thinks he's orange.
Skylar says she's tan.
Rhett says he's see-through.
"See, you can see how my veins are blue
but they're red when I bleed."

And I wish there was no such thing as springtime.
'Cause I don't trust the machines
that will one day be planting seeds in these gardens
teaching them that some people are flowers
some people are weeds,
rip the weeds by their roots
ignore their screams
tilt your own face to the sun
take what you want,
you are the chosen ones.

I wanna tell Jesse that Sitting Bull was wrong
when he said that white people are liars and thieves.

I wanna tell her we didn't come like a time bomb,
gunpowder on our breath,
teeth built like bullets,
that this land didn't weep when our feet
first mercilessly hit the ground.
I don't wanna say we drowned and maimed the children,
sliced long strips of their skin for bridle reigns.
I don't wanna say the moon was slain,
the constellations dispersed like shrapnel.
Jesse, mothers killed their babies, then killed themselves
when they saw our faces on the horizon
and all that we left was a trail of tears.

But if I have to say that
I wanna say our boats stopped there.
I wanna say the waves never saw the sails of slave ships,
never heard the sound of chain links,
but Jesse, think slaughterhouse.
Think people branded, suffocating, foaming at the mouth.
Can you imagine what kind of pain you would have to endure
to throw yourself overboard 1200 miles out to sea?

Lungs gratefully exchanging breath for saltwater,
gratefully trading life for death.

Can you imagine being chained to your dead daughter?
How many days would it take you to stop
searching her hands for lifelines?
To stop searching her fingertips for memories of sunshine?
To stop searching her wrists for a pulse,
for just some sign of time turning backwards
to when you just knew
people would never do things like this?

And Jesse this
is not just a picture our history,
not just a picture of our past.
We've been hundreds of years
measuring the size of their hearts
by the size of our fists,
erecting our bliss on the broken backs of dark skin.
The present is far from gift-wrapped.

Ask mothers in the Bronx
chasing rats out of their babies' cribs.
Ask the fathers of the kids
whose lives we exchange for cheap gas.
Ask our prisons why jail bars always come in black.
Ask the woman in Thailand whose cancer builds our laptops.
Ask the Mexican man working in a field fertilized by nerve gas.
Ask his daughter when she's born without fingers
or hands to pray with.
(ask me how long I could keep going with this list)
God might be watching,
but we are not.

You are white, Jesse.
There are bodies dangling
from the limbs of your family tree.
Our people pull people from their soil like weeds.
Breathe in our story.
Force yourself to hold it in your lungs
'til you can hear our hymns sung beneath white sheets.
Feel yourself fire as they shout.
Do not look away as bullet enters heartbeat.
Now breathe out.
This is where we come from.
This is still where we are.
Now, where will we go from here?

I don't believe we're hateful.
I think we're just asleep.
But when we wake we can't call up the dead and say,
"Sorry, we were looking the other way."

There are names and faces behind our apathy,
eulogies beneath our choices.
There are voices deep as roots
thundering unquestionable truth
through the white noise that pacifies our ears.
Don't tell me we can't hear.
Don't tell me we don't hear.
When the moon is slain,
when the constellations disperse like shrapnel,
don't you think it's time
something changed?

EVERY MONTH

Every month when I get my period
I breathe a sigh of relief and thank god I'm not pregnant,

'cause you never know when Jesus is coming back
and you never know who god's gonna choose
to be the next Virgin Mary

and can you imagine anything more scary
than staring down between your legs
and seeing the little glowing head of baby Jesus?
Holy shit, no thank you.

I mean, what kind of bumper sticker would you get?
'Your son's an honor student? Yeah well,
my son walks on water and heals lepers motherfuckers!'

Think of the pressure.
Personally I'd prefer to give birth to Lucifer,

a fixer-upper, the kind of kid who would sit at the last supper
and complain that Peter got more mashed potatoes,

'cause god knows
the holy have done more damage to this world
than the devil ever could.

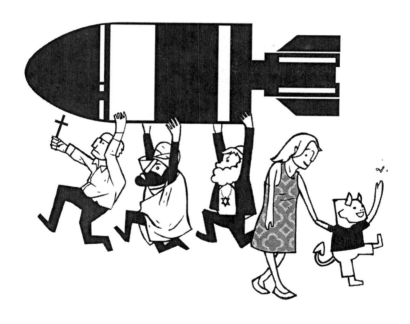

THE MOON IS A KITE

From the other end of the phone line
my little sister says, "Andrea, poppy flowers are beautiful."

I say, "You're right."
And I want to say,
"and landmines look like toys to children
until their limbs explode,
and their families find their bodies
in ditches on the side of the road."

Our mother is crying herself to sleep again tonight.
Your daughter is in my arms wondering where you are.
In the morning the sunbeams will look like jail bars.

Please come back.
Please.
I'll breathe *I love you* into your bloodstream
until the needles can't compare.
I'll tether my veins into thread
and stitch them through your torn seams.
I'll scream *LIGHT* into your bruises,
still lives beneath your track marks.
You can stand on the cliff of my heart
and shout nothing but ugly through me
I promise all I will echo back is
"Beauty, beauty, you have always been beauty."

Did I ever tell you on the day you were born
I stopped believing in Jesus
and started believing in You?
And sometimes it's the metal in the wind chimes

that reminds us how soft the breeze is.
So even when you grew like a switchblade,
pupils dilating the apocalypse,
more junk in your veins than blood,
more rage on your lips than love,
I still believed in you.

I knew you blew this world a kiss
and no one blew it back
and I wish I had a roadmap
back to that time before the first time
you mainlined midnight in search of an escape.
I wish I'd had your back that night.
I wish I'd told you, "Life is gonna hold you at gunpoint,
but time usually comes with a white flag."
'Cause right now there's a body bag around the sky
and every time your daughter cries
I see chalk outlines of crucified angels,

and I'm not sure I'm strong enough for this.
I can see the veins in my wrists too clearly
we're more alike than you know,
but your daughter's heart is beating.
I can see her pulse in the soft spot
on the top of her head.
In the other room our mother is asleep and dreaming now
of the way we were when we too were just babies like her,
and maybe we'll never be that new again.

Maybe there will always be days when the sunbeams look like jail bars.
Maybe it will seem we have more scars than lifelines sometimes,
but I've found it's always worth trying to find a way
to walk away from the land mines
and hope you come back
with your skin intact enough to drink the moonshine, girl.

I know you think this world is too dark to even dream in color,
but I've seen flowers bloom at midnight.
I've seen kites fly in gray skies
and they were real close to looking like the sunrise,
and sometime it takes the most wounded wings
the most broken things
to notice how strong the breeze is,
how precious the flight.

So I'm still not believing in Jesus.
I'm still believing in You.
I'm still telling your daughter,
"The moon is a kite
attached to a string
that's held by your mother
and I promise she's coming back soon."

EL MOZOTE

El Salvador, 1981.
In the village of El Mozote
the twilight sun was falling slow
behind the mountain's red earth.
December soil giving birth
to the stretching necks of noble pines, rising
falling shedding humble shadows upon the golden corn fields below

but the day's tender glow told nothing
of the dark fear of the people
hiding horrified in their homes.
And then the soldiers came.

The soldiers came in the name of cleansing,
cleansing their country free
of potential communist rebels.
Plan was, if they couldn't catch the fish
then they were gonna drain the sea.
So they pounded on the village doors
with the butts of their M16s,
"Get out here now!"
'til every person in the village was mouth-down in the dirt.

And the soldiers shouted questions
while mothers trembled and the children cried
and the fathers begged for their lives,
begged for their families to live, "We are an innocent people,
we have not taken sides, we have no answers to give."

And they had no answers to give.
So when night dropped its ebony skirt

the people of El Mozote were still
mouth-down in the dirt.
And there had never been a night so long,
sleepless with terror, the darkness drew on and on
so when dawn finally sprinkled her first shards of light
the people of the village
having lived through the night
dared, for a moment, hope.
But no.

The slaughter began with the men.
Fathers, brothers, grandfathers, sons,
not one was left alive.
Beheaded with machetes, their crimson corpses
were stacked and stacked and stacked in piles,
while each mother clutched her child to her chest
praying, "Jesus save us, Jesus save us."
They couldn't imagine the terror coming next.

The children were hung from trees,
tossed in the air and caught
on the bloodied blades of bayonets.
The women were slaughtered with M16s,
as their ten-year-old daughters
writhed in heaving pain beneath the soldiers' brutal sex,
their screams futile as the soft seams of their flesh
tore and ripped to fit the gang-raping warheads
of a sin no god would ever forgive.

And there has never been a sound more terrible,
more impossibly unbearable
than the desperate shrill of the death
piercing hour after hour the miles of El Salvador's hills,
and still, beneath it all,
like breath rises from shattered chests
and wings rise from burning nests

beneath it all
one little girl sang.

Through the slaughter of her father
and the slaughter of her mother,
a day howling a horror like no other
she sang.

As solider after soldier drilled her body
with his phallic hate,
she sang through rape after rape after brutal rape,
as everything around her bled desperate with cries
the little girl sang hymns to the sky.
She sang 'til they shot her in the chest,
and still she sang like the blessed of the blessed.
She sang 'til they shot her again
and even then as she choked on her blood she sang.
She sang 'til they slit her throat.

And she was only one of over 900 innocent people
tortured and killed that day at the massacre at El Mozote,
funded by the USA.
A crime covered up and denied by our government for years
because the killers were trained
in the School of the Americas, Ft. Benning, Georgia.

And now as the militia of the red, white, and blue
treads the guilty waters of another bloody slaughter
our nation's government is still hiding
still denying its people honest information.
But we who walk among the land of the relatively free
have an obligation to hunt down the truth,
have an obligation to lift our voices against any more pain
inflicted on anyone in our names.

Our resistance is the key.

The caged bird sings.
The caged bird would rather be free.

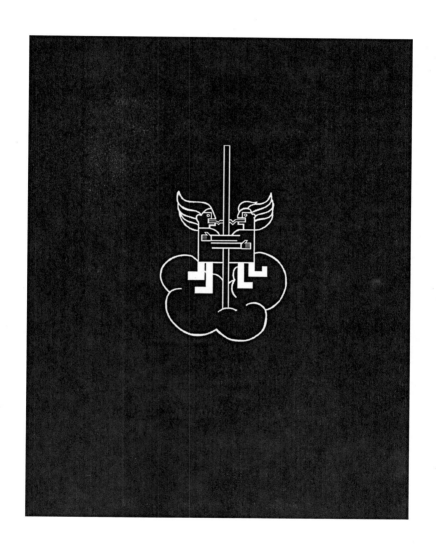

WHEN THE BOUGH BREAKS

It's two a.m.
The emergency room psychiatrist looks up from his clipboard
with eyes paid to care
and asks me if I see people who "aren't really there."
I say, "I see people...
how the hell am I supposed to know
if they're *really there* or not?"

He doesn't laugh.
Neither do I.
The math's not on my side,
ten stitches and one lie, "I swear I wasn't trying to die,
I just wanted to see what my pulse looked like from the inside."

Fast forward one year.
I'm standing in an auditorium behind a microphone
reading a poem to four hundred Latino high school kids
who live with the breath of the INS
crawling up their mothers' backbones
and I am frantically hiding my scars,
'cause the last thing I want these kids to know
is that I ever thought my life was too hard.

I've never seen a bomb drop.
I've never felt hunger.
I've also never seen lightning strike
but I know we've all heard the thunder
and it doesn't take a genius to tell something's burning.

"Please call me by my true name,
I am the child in Uganda all skin and bone."

Do we remember the rest?
And, "Jesus Wept."
Jesus wept, but look at our eyes,
dry as the desert sand
dusting the edges of our soldiers' wedding bands.

Do you know children in Palestine fly kites
to prove they're still free?
Can you imagine how that string
must feel between their fingers
as they kneel in the cinders of US-made missile heads?
You can count the dead by the colors in the sky.

The bough is breaking.
The cradle is falling.
Right now a six-year-old girl is crouched in a ditch in Lebanon
wishing on falling bombs.

Right now our government is recording the test scores
of Black and Latino 4th graders
to see how many prison beds will be needed in the year 2015.

Right now there's a man on the street outside my door
with outstretched hands full of heartbeats no one can hear.
He has cheeks like torn sheet music
every tear-broken crescendo falling on deaf ears.
At his side there's a boy with eyes like an anthem
no one stands up for.

Doctor, our insanity is not that we see people who aren't there.
It's that we ignore the ones who are.
'Til we find ourselves scarred and ashamed
walking into emergency rooms at two am
flooded with a pain we cannot name or explain,
bleeding from the outside in.
Our skin is not impervious.

Cultures built on greed and destruction
do not pick and choose who they kill.

Do we really believe our need for Prozac
has nothing to do with Fallujah,
with Kabul, with the Mexican border,
with the thousands of US school kids
bleeding budget cuts that will never heal
to fuel war tanks?

Thank god for denial.
Thank god we can afford the makeup
to pile upon the face of it all.
Look at the pretty world.
Look at all the smiling people,
and the sky with a missile between her teeth
and a steeple through her heart
and not a single star left to hold her

and the voices of a thousand broken nations
saying, "Wake me, wake me
when the American dream is over."

EAR MUFFS

My favorite teacher once told me
she wears three hats at the same time
while walking through her neighborhood
in the backwoods of Maine;
one to keep her head warm,
one to block the sun from her face,
and one bright orange hat
to keep the hunters from shooting her in the brain.

She looked at me seriously and said,
"I suppose I could get a hat that does all three
but that would be an awfully funny looking hat."

You, my love
are a funny looking hat.

That is to say,
you are everything I need.

Forgive me for the days
I am ear muffs
in Florida
on a sandy beach
during a heat wave.

SAY YES

When two violins are placed in a room
if a chord on one violin is struck
the other violin will sound the note.
If this is your definition of hope,
this is for you.
For the ones who know how powerful we are,
who know we can sound the music in the people around us
simply by playing our own strings.
For the ones who sing life into broken wings,
open their chests and offer their breath
as wind on a still day when nothing seems to be moving
spare those intent on proving god is dead.
For you when your fingers are red
from clutching your heart so it will beat faster.
For the time you mastered the art
of giving yourself for the sake of someone else.
For the ones who have felt what it is to crush the lies
and lift truth so high the steeples bow to the sky.

This is for you.

This is also for the people who wake early
to watch flowers bloom.
Who notice the moon at noon on a day when the world
has slapped them in the face with its lack of light.
For the mothers who feed their children first
and thirst for nothing when they're full.

This is for women.
And for the men who taught me
only women bleed with the moon,

but there are men who cry when women bleed
men who bleed from women's wounds.
And this is for that moon
on the nights she seems hung by a noose,
for the people who cut her loose
and for the people still waiting for the rope to burn
about to learn they have scissors in their hands.

This is for the man who showed me
the hardest thing about having nothing
is having nothing to give,
who said the only reason to live is to give ourselves away.
So this is for the day we'll quit or jobs
and work for something real.
We'll feel for sunshine in the shadows,
look for sunrays in the shade.
This is for the people who rattle the cage that slave wage built,
and for the ones who didn't know the filth until tonight
but right now are beginning songs that sound something like
people turning their porch lights on
and calling the homeless back home.

This is for all the shit we own,
and for the day we'll learn how much we have
when we learn to give that shit away.
This is for doubt becoming faith,
for falling from grace and climbing back up.
For trading our silver platters for something that matters,
like the gold that shines from our hands
when we hold each other.

This is for your grandmother,
who walked a thousand miles on broken glass
to find that single patch of grass to plant a family tree
where the fruit would grow to laugh.
For the ones who know the math of war

has always been subtraction
so they live like an action of addition.
For you when you give like every star is wishing on you,
and for the people still wishing on stars
this is for you too.

This is for the times you went through hell
so someone else wouldn't have to.
For the time you taught a 14-year-old girl
she was powerful.
For the time you taught a 14-year-old boy
he was beautiful.
For the radical anarchist asking a republican to dance,
'cause what's the chance of anyone moving from right to left
if the only moves they see are NBC and CBS.
This is for the no becoming yes,
for fear becoming trust,
for saying *I love you* to people who will never say it to us.

For scraping away the rust and remembering how to shine.
For the dime you gave away when you didn't have a penny,
For the many beautiful things we do,
for every song we've ever sung,
for refusing to believe in miracles
because miracles are the impossible coming true
and everything is possible.

This is for the possibility that guides us
and for the possibilities still waiting to sing
and spread their wings inside us,
'cause tonight Saturn is on his knees
proposing with all of his ten thousand rings
that whatever song we've been singing we sing even more.
The world needs us right now more than it ever has before.
Pull all your strings.
Play every chord.

If you're writing letters to the prisoners
start tearing down the bars.
If you're handing out flashlights in the dark
start handing out stars.

Never go a second hushing the percussion of your heart.
Play loud.
Play like you know the clouds
have left too many people cold and broken
and you're their last chance for sun.
Play like there's no time for hoping brighter days will come.
Play like the apocalypse is only 4...3...2... but you
have a drum in your chest that could save us.

You have a song like a breath that could raise us
like the sunrise into a dark sky that cries to be blue.
Play like you know we won't survive if you don't
but we will if you do.
Play like Saturn is on his knees
proposing with all of his ten thousand rings
that we give every single breath.
This is for saying, *YES*.
This is for saying, *YES*.

I DO

(sung)
ba bi di ba ba bi di ba ba ba bi ba bi di ba
ba dang a dang dang a dingy dong ding
I do I do I do
dip da dip da dip
I do I do
dip da dip da dup
ba bi di ba ba bi di ba ba ba bi ba bi di b
ba dang a dang dang a dingy dong ding

I do.........

But the fuckers say we can't.

'Cause you're a girl
and I'm a girl... or at least something close
so the most we can hope for
is an uncivil union in Vermont
and I want church bells.
I want rosary beads.
I want Jesus on his knees.
I wanna walk down the aisle
feeling the patriarchy smile.

That's not true.

But I do
wanna spend my life with you.
And I wanna know, fifty years from now,
when you're in a hospital room getting ready to die,
when visiting hours are for family members only,

I wanna know they'll let me in
to say goodbye.

'Cause I've been fifty years
memorizing the way the lines beneath your eyes
form rivers when you cry,
and I've held my hand like an ocean at your cheek
saying, "Baby, flow to me…"
'cause for fifty years I've watched you grow with me.

Fifty years of you never letting go of me
through nightmares and dreams
and everything in-between,
from the day I said, "Buy me a ring.
Buy me a ring that will turn my finger green
so I can imagine our love is a forest.
I wanna get lost in you."

And I swear I grew like a wild flower
every hour of the fifty years I was with you.
And that's not to say we didn't have hard days.
Like the day you said, "That check-out clerk was so sweet."
And I said, "I'd like to eat that check-out clerk."
And you said, "Honey, that's not funny."
And I said, "Baby, maybe you could take a fucking joke
every now and then."

So I slept on the couch that night.

But when morning came you were laughing.
Yeah, there were times we were both half-in
and half-out the door, but I never needed more

than the stars on your skin to lead me home.
For fifty years you were my favorite poem.
And I'd read you every night

knowing I might never understand every word
but that was ok 'cause the lines of you
were the closest thing to holy I'd ever heard.
You'd say, "This kind of love has to be verb.
We are paint on a slick canvas.
It's gonna take a whole lot to stick,
but if we do we'll be a masterpiece."

And we were.

From the beginning living in towns
that frowned at our hand-holding,
folding their stares like hate notes into our pockets
so we could pretend they weren't there.
You said, "Fear is only a verb if you let it be.
Don't you dare let go of my hand."
That was my favorite line.

That and the time when we saw two boys

kissing on the street in Kansas,
and we both broke down crying,
'cause it was Kansas and you said,
"What are the chances of seeing
anything but corn in Kansas!?"

We were born again that day.
I cut your cord and you cut mine
and the chords of time
played like a concerto of faith ,
like we could feel the rope unwind,
the fraying red noose of hate loosening,
loosening from years of…
People like you aren't welcome here.
People like you can't work here.
People like you cannot adopt.

So we had lots of cats and dogs
and once even a couple of monkeys
you taught to sing,
hey, hey we're the monkeys
You were crazy like that.

And I was so crazy about you
on nights you couldn't sleep
I'd lay awake for hours counting sheep for you,
and you would rewrite the rhythm of my heartbeat
with the way you held me in the morning,
resting your head on my chest
I swear my breath turned silver the day your hair did.
Like I swore marigolds grew
in the folds of my eyelids the first time saw you,
and they bloomed the first time I watched you
dance to the tune of our kitchen kettle in our living room.

In a world that could have left us hard as metal
we were soft as nostalgia together.
For fifty years we feathered wings too wide to be prey
and we flew through days strong and days fragile.
You would fold your love into an origami firefly
and throw it through my passageways
'til all my hidden chambers were lit with lanterns.
Now every trap door
of every pore of my body is open
because of you, because of us
so I do, I do, I do
wanna be in that room with you.

When visiting hours are for family members only
I wanna know they'll let me in.
I wanna know they'll let me hold you
while I sing…

ba bi di ba ba bidiba babi di ba bi di ba ba
dang a dang dang a dingy dong ding
I'm so in love with you
baby, I'm so in love with you
dip a dip a dip ba bi di ba a dang a dang dang
a dingy dong ding

good bye.

NOTES AND CREDITS

For Eli
Inspired by the shared letters of Eli Wright and his mother Vrnda dasi. I am forever grateful to both of them for their time and heart. For more info go to: www.LiberateThis.com and www.MFSO.org.

See-through
Much of the poem was inspired by Derrick Jensen's *The Culture of Make Believe*, Chelsea Green Publishing.

Titanic
170 degrees is not an exaggeration. Read *Dying to Cross: the Worst Immigrant Tragedy in American History*, by Jorge Ramos, Harper Collins.

ABOUT THE AUTHOR

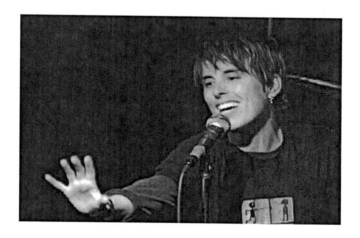

Rousing audiences internationally with her poignant message and her genuine interest in generating change, Andrea Gibson is a queer poet/activist whose work deconstructs the foundations of the current political machine, highlighting issues such as patriarchy, gender norms, white-supremacy and capitalist culture. Cementing her niche in the upper echelon of the national performance poetry slam scene, Andrea has placed in the top four on five international finals stages and was the first ever Women of the World Slam Champion in 2008. As a touring artist, Andrea has headlined everywhere from the Nuyorican Poet's Café, to Pride Fests and Lady Fests, to high schools and universities throughout the U.S. and Europe. She has been showcased on Free Speech TV, the BBC, the documentary "Slam Planet" and Independent Radio Stations worldwide. She currently a member of Vox Feminista, a multi-passionate performance tribe of radical, political performers bent on social change through cultural revolution. Andrea is an independent artist who has selfreleased three CD's, *Bullets and Windchimes*, *Swarm*, & *When the Bough Breaks*.

NEW FROM WRITE BLOODY BOOKS

EVERYTHING IS EVERYTHING (2010)
New poems by Cristin O'Keefe Aptowicz

DEAR FUTURE BOYFRIEND (2010)
A Write Bloody reissue of Cristin O'Keefe Aptowicz's first book of poetry

HOT TEEN SLUT (2010)
A Write Bloody reissue of Cristin O'Keefe Aptowicz's second book of poetry about her time writing for porn

WORKING CLASS REPRESENT (2010)
A Write Bloody reissue of Cristin O'Keefe Aptowicz's third book of poetry

OH, TERRIBLE YOUTH (2010)
A Write Bloody reissue of Cristin O'Keefe Aptowicz's fourth book of poetry about her terrible youth

CATACOMB CONFETTI (2010)
New poems by Josh Boyd

THE BONES BELOW (2010)
New poems by Sierra DeMulder

CEREMONY FOR THE CHOKING GHOST (2010)
New poems by Karen Finneyfrock

MILES OF HALLELUJAH (2010)
New poems by Rob "Ratpack Slim" Sturma

RACING HUMMINGBIRDS (2010)
New poems by Jeanann Verlee

YOU BELONG EVERYWHERE (2010)
Road memoir and how-to guide for travelling artists

LEARN THEN BURN (2010)
Anthology of poems for the classroom. Edited by Tim Stafford and Derrick Brown.

OTHER WRITE BLOODY BOOKS

STEVE ABEE, GREAT BALLS OF FLOWERS (2009)
New poems by Steve Abee

SCANDALABRA (2009)
New poetry compilation by Derrick Brown

DON'T SMELL THE FLOSS (2009)
New Short Fiction Pieces By Matty Byloos

THE LAST TIME AS WE ARE (2009)
New poems by Taylor Mali

IN SEARCH OF MIDNIGHT: THE MIKE MCGEE HANDBOOK OF AWESOME (2009)
New poems by Mike McGee

ANIMAL BALLISTICS (2009)
New poems by Sarah Morgan

CAST YOUR EYES LIKE RIVERSTONES INTO THE EXQUISITE DARK (2009)
New poems by Danny Sherrard

SPIKING THE SUCKER PUNCH (2009)
New poems by Robbie Q. Telfer

THE GOOD THINGS ABOUT AMERICA (2009)
An illustrated, un-cynical look at our American Landscape. Various authors.
Edited by Kevin Staniec and Derrick Brown

THE ELEPHANT ENGINE HIGH DIVE REVIVAL (2009)
Anthology

THE CONSTANT VELOCITY OF TRAINS (2008)
New poems by Lea C. Deschenes

HEAVY LEAD BIRDSONG (2008)
New poems by Ryler Dustin

UNCONTROLLED EXPERIMENTS IN FREEDOM (2008)
New poems by Brian Ellis

POLE DANCING TO GOSPEL HYMNS (2008)
Poems by Andrea Gibson

CITY OF INSOMNIA (2008)
New poems by Victor D. Infante

WHAT IT IS, WHAT IT IS (2008)
Graphic Art Prose Concept book by Maust of Cold War Kids and author Paul Maziar

OVER THE ANVIL WE STRETCH (2008)
New poems by Anis Mojgani

NO MORE POEMS ABOUT THE MOON (2008)
NON-Moon poems by Michael Roberts

JUNKYARD GHOST REVIVAL (2008)
with Andrea Gibson, Buddy Wakefield, Anis Mojgani, Derrick Brown, Robbie Q,
Sonya Renee and Cristin O'Keefe Aptowicz

THE LAST AMERICAN VALENTINE:
ILLUSTRATED POEMS TO SEDUCE AND DESTROY (2008)
24 authors, 12 illustrators team up for a collection of non-sappy love poetry.
Edited by Derrick Brown

LETTING MYSELF GO (2007)
Bizarre god comedy & wild prose by Buzzy Enniss

LIVE FOR A LIVING (2007)
New poems by Buddy Wakefield

SOLOMON SPARROWS ELECTRIC WHALE REVIVAL (2007)
Poetry compilation by Buddy Wakefield, Anis Mojgani, Derrick Brown, Dan
Leamen & Mike McGee

I LOVE YOU IS BACK (2006)
Poetry compilation (2004-2006) by Derrick Brown

BORN IN THE YEAR OF THE BUTTERFLY KNIFE (2004)
Poetry anthology, 1994-2004 by Derrick Brown

SOME THEY CAN'T CONTAIN (2004)
Classic poetry compilation by Buddy Wakefield

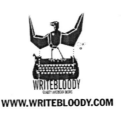

WWW.WRITEBLOODY.COM

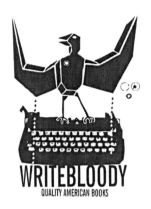

WRITEBLOODY
QUALITY AMERICAN BOOKS

PULL YOUR BOOKS UP BY THEIR BOOTSTRAPS

Write Bloody Publishing distributes and promotes great books of fiction, poetry and art every year. We are an independent press dedicated to quality literature and book design, with an office in Long Beach, CA.

Our employees are authors and artists so we call ourselves a family. Our design team comes from all over America: modern painters, photographers and rock album designers create book covers we're proud to be judged by.

We publish and promote 8-12 tour-savvy authors per year. We are grass-roots, D.I.Y., bootstrap believers. Pull up a good book and join the family. Support independent authors, artists and presses.

Visit us online:

writebloody.com

CPSIA information can be obtained
at www.ICGtesting.com
Printed in the USA
FFOW04n0621071213
2559FF